GUIDE THREE:
HEALTHY STYLING, STRONG HAIR

From Root to Tip: A Growing Hands Guide for Natural Hair

BY CONSTANCE HUNTER

For permissions, inquiries, or additional resources, please contact:

Pre'Vail Natural Hair Salon

www.prevailyournatural.com | prevailyournatural@gmail.com

This book is intended for informational and educational purposes only and should serve as a general guide to understanding and improving natural hair health. While the methods and recommendations provided are based on expertise in natural hair care and trichology, they are not intended to replace professional medical or dermatological advice.

If you are experiencing severe scalp conditions, excessive hair loss, or other persistent issues, it is strongly recommended that you consult a licensed dermatologist or a professional cosmetologist specializing in scalp and hair health. A trained professional can assess underlying causes and provide personalized treatment plans tailored to your specific needs.

By using the information in this book, the reader acknowledges that the author and publisher are not responsible for individual outcomes. Readers should exercise their own discretion when applying the suggested practices.

First Edition: 2025

ISBN:

Paperback: 978-1-968134-03-7

Ebook: 978-1-968134-12-9

Printed in USA

ABOUT THE AUTHOR

As a certified trichologist and natural hair care educator, I specialize in helping individuals discover what's truly possible for their hair—especially when they've been told otherwise.

My passion lies in witnessing transformation—that moment when someone realizes their hair can be healthy, strong, and free. With a deep understanding of the science behind hair and scalp health, I strive to provide clarity, comfort, and actionable solutions. My training equips me to assess and guide care for a wide range of concerns, from common challenges like dandruff and dryness to complex conditions such as alopecia areata, scalp psoriasis, and CCCA.

But my work goes beyond diagnosis or technique. I believe in education, empowerment, and helping clients build routines that nourish their crown from root to tip. This includes learning to read labels, choosing products with purpose, avoiding harmful styling practices, and embracing care that fits their lifestyle and values.

While I offer expert insight from the field of trichology, I'm not a medical doctor. Hair and scalp symptoms can sometimes signal deeper health issues. That's why I encourage a holistic approach—and, when necessary, consulting licensed healthcare professionals for comprehensive support.

In this series, you'll find guidance rooted in science, experience, and care. My hope is that it not only helps you understand your hair better but also love it more, trust it more, and grow with it in ways you never thought possible.

Your hair is not the problem—you just needed the right guide.

DEDICATION

For the one whose styles once came at the cost of her strands:

You don't have to choose between beauty and health—
you deserve both.

OVERVIEW

Styling your hair shouldn't mean sacrificing your strands. *Healthy Styling, Strong Hair* teaches you how to style with intention—protecting your hair's strength while celebrating its beauty.

Discover techniques that retain length, reduce tension, and allow your hair to flourish under your creativity.

Because your crown deserves styles that *support*—not stress—it.

SERIES INTRODUCTION

Welcome to *From Root to Tip: A Growing Hands Guide for Natural Hair*

This series was created with one goal in mind: to give you what's been missing—not just products, not just trends, but truth, support, and real guidance for real people who are ready to finally understand and care for their natural hair from the inside out.

For years, we've been taught to manage, fix, or fight our hair. But here, we're doing something different. We're returning to care—not control. To confidence. To consistency. To choice.

Each guide in this series is built as a step in your journey. They can be read in order or on their own, depending on where you are in your process. Whether you're just starting out, rebuilding your relationship with your hair, or deepening your understanding, this space is for you.

I've written these guides from my hands—growing hands that have touched, healed, protected, and restored countless crowns. Now, I offer that care to you.

This isn't just about hair. It's about healing. It's about reclaiming your rhythm, your confidence, and your beauty—from root to tip.

Let's begin.

WHAT YOU WILL LEARN

- What makes a style truly *protective*

- How to prep your hair for styling (trims, hydration, and detangling)

- Techniques for low-tension braids, twists, and updos

- How to protect your styles overnight with wraps, bonnets, and more

- The importance of proper takedown to prevent breakage

- Styling habits that align with your growth goals

WHAT YOU'LL WALK AWAY WITH

- A styling approach that supports retention—not setbacks

- Tips for balancing style, health, and ease

- Fewer breakage incidents and more consistent growth

- The confidence to style without fear of damage

TABLE OF CONTENTS

INTRODUCTION

It shouldn't hurt to look good.

In *Healthy Styling, Strong Hair*, we dive into styling methods that protect your hair from breakage, tension, and long-term damage. Whether you love braids, twists, buns, or heatless curls, this guide teaches you how to create styles that are both beautiful and safe.

From prep to takedown, night care to daily maintenance—you'll learn to make styling a part of your healthy hair plan, not the reason you have to start over.

LESSON 1:
PROTECTIVE STYLES

Protective styles are a crucial aspect of hair care for individuals with natural textured hair. These styles are designed to minimize manipulation and shield the hair from environmental damage, allowing it to grow and stay healthy. This lesson will explore different types of protective styles, their benefits, and the proper methods for installation and maintenance.

Types of Protective Styles and Their Benefits

1. Braids

Braids are among the most popular protective styles and come in a variety of forms, including box braids, cornrows, and Senegalese twists. Each type offers its own unique benefits:

- **Box Braids:** These individual plaits can be styled in various lengths and sizes. Box braids are versatile, allowing for everything from intricate patterns to simple, sleek styles. They protect the ends of the hair, reducing exposure to harsh elements and minimizing breakage.

- **Cornrows:** Cornrows are braids that lie flat against the scalp in straight, narrow rows. This style is excellent for protecting the scalp while keeping the hair neatly secured. Cornrows can also be adorned with beads, threads, or other accessories, adding a decorative touch to their protective function.

- **Senegalese Twists:** These rope-like twists are created using extensions or natural hair. They provide a smooth, shiny finish and can be worn in various lengths. Senegalese twists offer protection by keeping the hair in a low-manipulation state, which helps prevent breakage and tangling.

2. Buns and Updo's

Buns and updos involve gathering and securing the hair in one section of the head. They are effective for protecting hair from daily wear and tear and can be styled in various ways:

- **High Buns:** This style involves pulling the hair into a high, secure bun on top of the head. High buns reduce exposure to the elements and are ideal for preventing tangling and breakage.

- **Low Buns:** Low buns are positioned at the nape of the neck or lower on the head. They provide a more understated look while still offering protection to the ends of the hair.

- **Chignons and French Rolls:** These elegant styles are perfect for formal occasions and provide full protection to the hair. They involve rolling or tucking the hair in a sophisticated manner, shielding it from environmental damage.

3. Wigs and Weaves

Wigs and weaves are versatile protective styles that involve adding hair extensions to the natural hair. Proper installation and removal are crucial to prevent damage and breakage. These styles offer several benefits:

- **Wigs:** Wigs completely cover natural hair, giving it a chance to rest and recover. They can be styled in various ways, providing a break from daily styling and manipulation. Wigs also allow for experimentation with different looks without altering the natural hair.

- **Weaves:** Weaves involve sewing or bonding hair extensions to the natural hair, adding length, volume, and texture. Weaves protect the natural hair by keeping it braided or in a low- manipulation state underneath the extensions.

4. Twists and Loss

Twists and locs are protective styles that involve twisting the hair into various formations:

- **Two-Strand Twists:** These twists involve dividing the hair into two sections and twisting them around each other. Two-strand twists can be done with natural hair or with added extensions for extra length and volume. They are easy to maintain and protect the hair by minimizing manipulation.

- **Sister Locs and Traditional Locs:** Locs are formed by matting and locking sections of hair. Sister locs are smaller and more uniform, while traditional locs are thicker and less uniform. Both styles offer long-term protection by keeping the hair in a low-manipulation state and reducing exposure to harsh elements.

How to Properly Install and Maintain Protective Styles

1. Installation

Proper installation of protective styles is essential for maximizing their benefits and preventing damage. Protective styles should not be worn for more than 8 weeks at a time before a new prep is needed.

- **Preparation:** Begin by thoroughly cleansing and conditioning the hair to remove product buildup, ensuring a clean, healthy base. Gently detangle the hair to minimize breakage during the styling process. This is the time to prep your hair for protection, including completing any trims and/or deep conditioning treatments. Doing so will help prevent irritation during the no- touch period.

- **Sectioning:** Divide the hair into manageable sections. Blow-dry the hair on low to medium heat, ensuring the process is smokeless. Use clips or hair ties to keep sections separated. Proper sectioning ensures even distribution of extensions or braiding, contributing to a neat and secure style.

- **Technique:** Follow the specific technique required for your chosen style. For braids, ensure that each braid is tight but not too tight to avoid tension on the scalp. For wigs, ensure proper fitting and secure attachment to prevent slipping or discomfort.

- **Use Quality Products:** Use proper tools and high-quality products for installation, including extensions, braiding hair, or adhesives for wigs. Ensure that all products are gentle on the hair and scalp to prevent irritation and damage.

2. Maintenance

Maintaining protective styles involves regular care to ensure both the style and the natural hair underneath remain healthy. The prep work helps lock moisture into the hair for the duration of the style.

- **Scalp Care:** Keep the scalp clean and moisturized. Use a lightweight oil or grease to maintain hydration and prevent dryness. Gently massage the scalp to stimulate circulation and promote healthy hair growth.

- **Moisture Retention:** Continue moisturizing the natural hair while it is protected. Use a spray or leave-in conditioner to add moisture without disrupting the style. Avoid heavy products that may lead to buildup.

- **Avoid Excessive Manipulation:** Minimize manipulation of the protective style to prevent stress on the hair and scalp. Avoid pulling or tugging on the hair, as this can lead to breakage and scalp irritation. Be mindful of ponytail placement to avoid tightly securing the edges, which can help prevent perimeter breakage.

- **Protect at Night:** Use a satin or silk scarf, bonnet, or pillowcase to protect the style while sleeping. These materials reduce friction and moisture loss, which can otherwise lead to dryness and breakage.

- **Regular Checks:** Periodically check the style for signs of damage or discomfort. Ensure that the style is still secure and that there are no issues, such as tangling or tension. If any problems arise, remove the style promptly to prevent further damage. While some styles may last longer than 8 weeks, remember that the protection benefits stop at 8 weeks.

- **Removing Styles:** When it's time to remove the protective style, do so carefully to avoid damaging the natural hair. Gently unravel braids or twists, and remove wigs or weaves without pulling or tugging. Follow up with a thorough cleansing and conditioning routine to restore the hair's health and prepare it for the next style. A cleansing shampoo is not recommended after removal. Instead, rinse the hair thoroughly and shampoo with a moisturizing shampoo. I recommend using three shampoos instead of the usual two to ensure the hair is fully cleansed.

Protective styles are essential for maintaining the health and integrity of natural textured hair. By understanding the different types of protective styles and implementing proper installation and maintenance techniques, individuals can maximize the benefits of these styles, promote hair growth, and minimize damage. Whether opting for braids, buns, wigs, or locs, the key is to prioritize care and attention to ensure both the style and the natural hair underneath remain healthy and vibrant.

LESSON 2:
LOW HEAT AND HEAT-FREE STYLING

In the world of hair care, heat-free styling has gained popularity as a healthier approach, especially for those with natural textured hair. This technique avoids the use of heat tools like flat irons and curling wands, which can cause damage over time. Instead, it utilizes alternative methods to achieve beautiful and varied styles.

However, while heat-free styling may seem like a safer option, it can still cause damage if not done with proper precautions. Understanding that hair is at its weakest when wet is essential. Heat-free styling often involves processes like detangling, parting, and styling, which can increase the risk of breakage. For example, detangling brushes that spread like a hand can rip out hair. To avoid this, discontinue their use and invest in the FHI Unbrush, which is gentler and better suited for this method.

Techniques for Achieving Fabulous Styles Without Heat

Before starting any of these styles, use either the LOC (Liquid, Oil, Cream) or LCO (Liquid, Cream, Oil) method to lock in moisture and prepare the hair for styling.

1. Twist-Outs

Twist-outs are a popular and versatile heat-free styling method for creating defined curls and waves. This technique involves twisting sections of hair and allowing them to set before unraveling to reveal soft, bouncy curls.

How to Do It:

- Start with damp, detangled hair.

- Apply a leave-in conditioner or styling cream to each section of hair.

- Twist the sections tightly from root to tip.

- Allow the twists to air-dry completely (usually 24 to 48 hours—no dryers).

- Once dry, apply a light oil to your hands and gently unravel the twists using your fingers or a wide-tooth comb to maintain definition.

- Benefits: Twist-outs are excellent for achieving natural-looking curls without heat. They offer flexibility in styling, allowing you to create tight curls or loose waves depending on your preference.

2. Braid-Out

Braid-outs are similar to twist-outs but involve braiding the hair to achieve defined curls with a slightly different texture. This technique is ideal for adding volume and body to your hair.

How to Do It:

- Begin with damp hair and apply a styling product that enhances hold and definition.

- Divide the hair into small sections and braid each section securely but not too tightly.

- Let the braids air-dry completely (usually 24 to 48 hours—no dryers).

- Gently unravel the braids to reveal voluminous, well-defined curls.

Benefits: Braid-outs are great for creating fuller, more textured curls. They add body and movement to the hair, making them perfect for those seeking a voluminous look.

3. Flexi-Rod Sets

Flexi-rods are foam rollers that bend to secure hair in place, making them an excellent tool for creating curls and waves without heat. They are available in various sizes, allowing you to customize your curl pattern.

How to Do It: Apply a setting lotion or styling mousse to damp hair. Divide the hair into sections and wrap each section around a flexi-rod, rolling it up toward the scalp. Secure the rod by bending its ends. Allow the hair to air-dry naturally or sit under a hooded dryer for faster results. Once dry, gently remove the flexi-rods and use your fingers to separate the curls for added volume and definition.

Benefits: Flexi-rods create long-lasting curls with minimal damage. They are versatile, enabling you to achieve various curl sizes and styles, from tight ringlets to loose waves.

4. Perm Rod Sets

Perm rods are similar to flexi-rods but are made of harder plastic. Available in various sizes, they are used to create long-lasting curls and waves.

How to Do It: Start with damp hair and apply a styling mousse or a light moisturizer. Section the hair and wrap each section around a perm rod, rolling it up to the scalp and securing it with the rod's clip. Allow the hair to air-dry or use a hooded dryer. Once the hair is completely dry, carefully remove the perm rods and gently separate the curls for a defined, bouncy look. If the hair is not smooth on the roller, saturate it with more mousse or water—this may help achieve a sleeker result.

Benefits: Perm rods create tight, well-defined curls and offer versatile styling options. They are especially effective for those seeking long-lasting curl definition without relying on heat.

5. Bantu Knots

Bantu knots are a traditional African hairstyle that involves sectioning the hair, twisting it into small knots, and allowing it to set. This method produces beautifully defined curls with minimal heat.

How to Do It: Begin with damp, detangled hair. Apply a leave-in conditioner or styling cream, then section the hair and twist each section into a small knot close to the scalp. Secure each knot with a hair tie or bobby pin. Let the hair air-dry completely before unraveling the knots to reveal well-defined curls.

Benefits: Bantu knots are excellent for creating a unique, textured curl pattern. Additionally, this style is protective, as it keeps the hair's ends tucked away, reducing breakage.

Styling Preparation Tips

Regardless of the style, it's essential to properly prep the hair for daily wear. Always follow these steps:

1. Shampoo and condition the hair.
2. Apply a leave-in conditioner.
3. Use an oil to seal in moisture.
4. Blow-dry the hair, if needed.
5. Apply a styling product such as mousse or setting lotion.

A highly recommended option is Nairobi Wrapp-It Shine Foaming Lotion, which blends well with most product combinations and does not flake, ensuring smooth, polished results.

Recommended Products and Tools for Heat-Free Styling

1. Styling Products

- **Leave-In Conditioners:** Leave-in conditioners are essential for heat-free styling techniques like twist-outs and braid-outs. They provide moisture and detangling benefits, helping to keep hair manageable. Choose products that offer hold without leaving the hair stiff or crunchy for a natural, soft finish.

- **Curl Creams and Gels:** Curl creams and gels are ideal for defining curls and adding structure to heat-free styles. Opt for lightweight formulas with a flexible hold to maintain bouncy, natural-looking curls without weighing the hair down.

- **Setting Lotions:** Setting lotions are designed to help hair maintain its shape when using rollers or rods. They provide a firm hold, enhance curl definition, and minimize frizz, making them perfect for achieving polished, long-lasting styles.

2. Tools

- **Flexi-Rods:** Flexi-rods are versatile and come in various sizes, making them ideal for creating a range of curl patterns. Their flexibility allows for easy adjustment, ensuring a custom curl look that suits your style.

- **Perm Rods:** Perm rods are excellent for achieving well-defined and long-lasting curls. Available in different diameters, they work well on various hair lengths and are a must-have for structured styles.

- **Detangle Brush:** A detangle brush is crucial for smoothing and detangling hair before styling. It prevents breakage and ensures the hair is manageable. Avoid brushes that spread wide like a hand, as they can create excessive force during detangling, snapping hair strands and thinning out hair over time.

- **Silk or Satin Scarves:** Protect your hair while you sleep with a silk or satin scarf. These materials reduce friction, helping to maintain your style and minimize frizz. They also prevent moisture loss, keeping hair hydrated overnight.

- **Hooded Dryers:** While not entirely heat-free, hooded dryers can speed up the drying process for styles that need to set. They are less damaging than direct heat tools and can be used in moderation to safely achieve professional-looking results.

LESSON 3:
TIPS FOR ACHIEVING DELINED CURLS

Achieving and maintaining defined curls is a key goal for many individuals with naturally textured hair. Defined curls not only highlight the hair's natural beauty but also contribute to a polished and well-groomed appearance. In this lesson, we will explore various curl-enhancing methods and products, along with effective techniques for defining and maintaining natural curls.

While products can help enhance curl definition, moisture remains the most critical factor. It is challenging to achieve defined curls when hair is dry and damaged. Curly hair, due to its looser cuticles and tendency to shrink, struggles to retain its natural form once the cuticles are sealed with proteins and keratins. This moisture blockage can lead to brittleness.

Curl Enhancing Methods and Products

1. Curl Creams and Gels

Curl creams and gels are essential for defining curls and maintaining their shape. These products provide hold and structure while enhancing the natural curl pattern.

Curl Cream: These are formulated to hydrate and define curls without leaving them stiff or crunchy. Many contain moisturizing ingredients like shea butter, olive oil, or aloe vera, which help keep curls soft and manageable.

Application: Apply a generous amount of curl cream to damp hair, focusing on the ends. Use your fingers or a detangling brush to distribute the product evenly and encourage curl formation.

Curl Gels: Gels provide a firmer hold compared to creams, making them ideal for creating defined, bouncy curls. Choose alcohol-free gels to prevent dryness.

Application: Apply gel to wet hair and use techniques like the "finger coiling" method, a detangling brush, or scrunching to enhance curl definition. Let hair air-dry or use a diffuser attachment on a blow dryer for faster drying.

2. Leave-In Conditioners

Leave-in conditioners add moisture and aid in detangling, making them a valuable step in any curl-enhancing routine. They also help prepare hair for styling products, improving curl definition.

Application: Apply leave-in conditioner to damp hair, focusing on the mid-lengths and ends. This locks in moisture and creates a smooth base for styling products. Use a detangling brush or fingers to ensure even distribution.

3. Curl Activators

Curl activators are specifically designed to enhance the natural curl pattern and reduce frizz. These products often provide hold and definition without weighing the hair down. A popular option is Taliah Waajid Curly Curl Gello.

Application: Apply curl activator to wet hair using the "raking" method, working the product from root to tip. This technique helps separate and define individual curls. Let hair air-dry or use a diffuser to set the curls.

4. Hair Oils

Hair oils, such as argan oil, jojoba oil, and castor oil, add shine and reduce frizz. They also help lock in moisture, improving overall curl definition.

Application: After styling, apply a small amount of hair oil to your palms and gently scrunch it into your curls. This adds shine and helps separate and define curls. Be careful not to use too much oil, as it can weigh down the hair.

Techniques for Defining and Maintaining Natural Curls

1. The Shingling Method

The shingling method is a popular technique for defining curls and ensuring even product distribution.

How to Do It: Start with wet, detangled hair. Apply a curl cream or gel to a section of hair, then use your fingers to rake the product through from root to tip. This ensures every strand is coated, enhancing curl definition. Repeat the process on all sections of hair, then allow it to air- dry or use a diffuser for faster drying. If desired, mist hair with water after applying the product to make it more pliable. This can give you more defined, "popping" curls with any of these methods.

2. The Finger-Coiling Method

Finger-coiling is a technique used to create well-defined curls by individually twisting sections of hair around your fingers.

How to Do It: After applying a curl cream or gel, take a small section of hair and wrap it around your finger to form a curl. Hold for a few seconds, then release. Repeat this process on all sections of hair. Allow the hair to air-dry or use a hooded dryer. Once dry, gently separate the curls with your fingers to add volume and reduce clumping, or leave the curls as-is and let your pillow do the work while you sleep.

3. The Plopping Method

Plopping is a technique that involves using a T-shirt or microfiber towel to enhance curl definition and reduce frizz.

How to Do It: After applying styling products to wet hair, lay a T-shirt or microfiber towel flat on a surface. Bend forward and gently place your curls into the center of the fabric. Wrap the edges around your head and secure it, creating a "plop." Leave the hair to dry in this position for 20-30 minutes. This method helps maintain curl shape and reduce frizz.

4. Diffusing

A diffuser is an attachment for a blow dryer that helps enhance curl definition and reduce frizz while drying.

How to Do It: After applying curl products, attach the diffuser to your blow dryer. Flip your head upside down or tilt it to one side, then gently place the diffuser under sections of hair. Use a low or medium heat setting and move the diffuser in a circular motion to dry your curls. This technique adds volume and reduces frizz.

5. Pineapple Technique

The pineapple technique is a method used to protect curls while sleeping and maintain their definition.

How to Do It: Gather your hair into a loose, high ponytail on top of your head using a silk or satin scrunchie. This helps preserve the curl pattern and prevents tangling. Cover your hair with a silk or satin scarf or bonnet to reduce friction and moisture loss. In the morning, gently release the ponytail and shake your head to separate the curls for a refreshed look.

6. Regular Trims

Regular trims are essential for maintaining healthy curls and preventing split ends, which can affect curl definition.

How to Do It: Schedule trims every 6-8 weeks to remove split ends and maintain the shape of your curls. Trim only the ends to preserve length while keeping your curls defined and healthy.

7. Hydration and Conditioning

Maintaining hydration and conditioning is crucial for keeping curls defined and preventing dryness.

Hydration: Use a moisturizing shampoo and conditioner to keep curls hydrated. Deep condition regularly for extra moisture and improved curl elasticity.

Conditioning: Incorporate leave-in conditioners and hair masks into your routine to provide ongoing moisture and nourishment. This keeps curls soft, manageable, and well-defined.

8. Avoiding Over-Manipulation

Excessive handling of your curls can lead to frizz and disrupt their definition.

How to Do It: Minimize touching and styling your hair throughout the day. Instead, focus on setting your curls using the techniques mentioned above, then allow them to air-dry or set naturally.

Product Recommendations

1. **Curl Creams:** Look for curl creams that offer moisture, hold, and frizz control. Popular options include SheaMoisture Curl Enhancing Smoothie and DevaCurl Super Cream.

2. **Curl Gels:** Opt for alcohol-free gels that provide flexible hold. Excellent choices include EcoStyle Argan and Black Castor Oil Gel and Design Essentials Almond Avocado Defining Creme Gel.

3. **Leave-In Conditioners:** Consider leave-in conditioners that provide hydration and detangling benefits, such as Paul Mitchell The Conditioner and Design Essentials Almond Avocado Detangling Leave-In Conditioner.

4. **Curl Activators:** Curl activators like Taliah Waajid Curly Curl Gello or Roux BIG POPPA Defining Gel are great for enhancing curl definition.

5. **Hair Oils:** Use lightweight oils like argan oil, jojoba oil, or castor oil to add shine and reduce frizz. Argan oil, in particular, is highly beneficial for its moisturizing properties.

By incorporating these techniques and products into your hair care routine, you can achieve and maintain beautifully defined curls that highlight the natural beauty of your textured hair.

QUIZ
HAIR STYLING TECHNIQUES

Lesson 1: Protective Styles

1. Question

Which of the following is considered a protective style?

a) Loose hair with daily combing.

b) Box braids.

c) Daily heat styling.

d) Hair extensions without moisturizing.

Answer: b) Box braids.

2. Question

What is the primary benefit of protective styles for natural hair?

a) It allows for frequent hair washing.

b) It prevents damage from environmental factors and manipulation.

c) It promotes faster hair growth in all cases.

d) It makes hair more manageable for daily styling.

Answer: b) It prevents damage from environmental factors and manipulation

3. Question

Which of the following is a best practice when maintaining protective styles?

a) Leaving the style in for more than 3 months without maintenance.

b) Avoiding any moisture or oil to keep the style intact.

c) Moisturizing the scalp regularly.

d) Constantly re-tightening the style to maintain tension.

Answer: c) Moisturizing the scalp regularly.

Lesson 2: Heat-Free Styling

1. Question

What is a recommended heat-free styling method for natural hair?

a) Using a curling iron on low heat.

b) Applying heat protectant before using flat irons.

c) Bantu knots or twist-outs.

d) Blowing hair dry on a high heat setting.

Answer: c) Bantu knots or twist-outs.

2. Question

Which tool is commonly used for heat-free curling of natural hair?

a) Flat iron.

b) Curling wand.

c) Flexi rods.

d) Hair dryer with diffuser.

Answer: c) Flexi rods.

3. Question

Which of the following is a benefit of heat-free styling?

a) Reduces the need for moisturizers.

b) Prevents heat damage.

c) Results in faster styling times.

d) Increases the frequency of hair washing.

Answer: b) Prevents heat damage.

Lesson 3: Tips for Achieving Defined Curls

1. Question

What is a key technique for achieving defined curls in natural hair?

a) Using a heavy oil before applying curl cream.

b) Detangling hair completely prior to styling.

c) Brushing dry hair with a fine-tooth comb.

d) Applying products to completely dry hair for better hold.

Answer: b) Detangling hair completely prior to styling.

2. Question

Which of the following products is commonly used to define natural curls?

a) Leave-in conditioner.

b) Curl defining gel or cream.

c) Clarifying shampoo.

d) Deep conditioner.

Answer: b) Curl defining gel or cream.

3. Question

a) What method helps to maintain curl definition overnight?

b) Using a hair straightener before bed.

c) Pineapple method or sleeping with a satin scarf.

d) Brushing the hair into a tight ponytail.

e) Applying a hair mask and leaving it in overnight.

Answer: b) Pineapple method or sleeping with a satin scarf.

4. Question

Which hair care technique helps with curl longevity throughout the day?

a) Applying curl products to dry hair only.

b) Refreshing curls with a water-based mist or leave-in spray.

c) Using hairspray immediately after washing.

d) Brushing through curls to keep them defined.

Answer: b) Refreshing curls with a water-based mist or leave-in spray.

CLOSING NOTE

Your strands don't have to suffer for your style.

This is your permission to slay *and* stay strong—because healthy hair *is* stylish hair.

www.ingramcontent.com/pod-product-compliance
Lightning Source LLC
Chambersburg PA
CBHW070259290326
41930CB00041B/2652